Boundless Energy

====================

*Discover How to Boost Energy
Levels Naturally So You Can Get
More Done, Feel Less Stressed and
Live Life to the Max*

RON KNESS

Contents

Disclaimer

This book has been written for information purposes only. Every effort has been made to make this book as complete and accurate as possible. However, there may be mistakes in typography or content. Also, this book provides information only up to the publishing date. Therefore, this book should be used as a guide - not as the ultimate source.

The purpose of this book is to educate. The author and the publisher does not warrant that the information contained in this book is fully complete and shall not be responsible for any errors or omissions. The author and publisher shall have neither liability nor responsibility to any person or entity with respect to any loss or damage caused or alleged to be caused directly or indirectly by this book.

Introduction

Everyone is always talking about time management. There just aren't enough hours in the day for many of us and so the belief goes that if we could squeeze a little more productivity out of our time, we'd be able to accomplish our dreams, earn more money, stay more organized *and* enjoy more time off.

It all sounds great, except for one thing: the entire endeavor is completely misguided. Sounds harsh but in fact it's also completely *true*. Your problem is not with time. You have *plenty* of time. If you didn't have plenty of time, you probably wouldn't have been 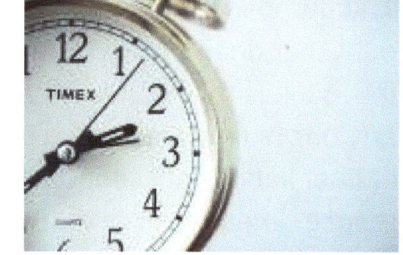 able to watch that entire boxset of Criminal Minds Season 10 would you? And you likely wouldn't have spent so long on YouTube...

The problem isn't time – it's energy. Your energy, just like your time, is finite. Only it actually exists in somewhat smaller quantities meaning that it's all too easy to run out and end up completely exhausted. And *that's* when we start to use our time poorly and not get much done.

Think about it: imagine if you could jump out of bed feeling energetic first thing in the morning. What would you do with that extra hour of productivity? Hit the gym maybe? Make some calls? Do last night's washing up so that you could live in a house that wouldn't *always* be untidy?

Remember when you were a little kid and you could just run around all day without ever seeming to get tired? Wouldn't it be incredible if you could get that back?

That's what we'll be looking at in this book…

So what will you learn in this e-book specifically? Here are just some of the topics we'll be covering:

- How to assess your own energy levels

- How mitochondrial function contributes to your energy levels and how to get back the mitochondrial function you had in your youth

- How to use supplements to give yourself a 'competitive edge' when it comes to energy

- How to choose superfoods that supercharge your energy

- How to avoid foods that drain your energy and slow your body down

- What type of training you can use to increase your energy

- The role of stress in energy management

- The secrets to a perfect night's sleep and how this leads to enhanced energy

- How habits and morning schedule contribute to your energy

- How more energy makes you perform better – and even be smarter!

- And much more!

Has Fatigue Deteriorated Your Quality of Life?

To start with then, let us assess how your potentially low energy levels may already be affecting your lifestyle. Does your energy need an upgrade? Or are already operating on 'full'?

Well let's take a look at the facts. Unless you're some kind of energy guru/prodigy, it's a fair bet that you already have chronically low energy. Why? Because it's a fact that *most* people are stressed. Specifically, nearly half of adults report feeling stressed every day. 44% of Americans report feeling more stressed year on year and work-related stress reportedly causes 10% of strokes.

We *know* that stress leads to adrenal fatigue and low energy, so statistically, you're likely to already be experiencing low energy.

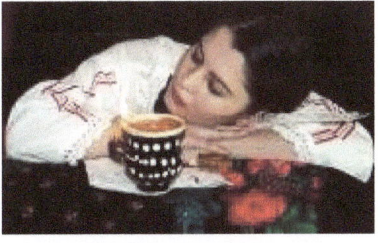

What's more, low testosterone is also a statistical likelihood if you're a man. Testosterone prescriptions have doubled in the last ten years and one in forty men over 30 have 'low testosterone'. Bearing in mind that this 'low testosterone' is measured against an *already very low* level that is considered acceptable. Mankind has far less testosterone in the modern age owing to stress, owing to xenoestrogens in the water, owing to less physical activity – and guess what? Low testosterone is *also* a cause of low energy. Seeing a pattern?

Vitamin D is also chronically low in most of the population. This also causes low energy. Other common vitamin deficiencies that *most* people suffer from at some point include low vitamin B12, low magnesium, low iron... they *all* lead to low energy.

So yes, chances are that you have 'low energy' – even if you're no less energetic than your colleagues and friends. Remember that little kid version of you who used to run around the house all day? *That's* what great energy should look like!

And of course there's a chance that you might be even *lower* on energy than this already-low norm...

Signs That You May be Low on Energy

Here are just some signs that your energy levels might be low...

- You find it difficult to get up in the morning

- You feel emotionally exhausted, stressed or depressed

- You find it hard to focus on work

- You find it hard to stay motivated by work

- Your career is suffering

- Your libido is low

- The house is untidy because you can't muster the energy to tidy it

- Your evenings are wasted

- You don't feel like going out

- You can't commit to a training program or a healthy diet plan

If any of these things sound familiar, then your quality of life is suffering due to a lack of energy. If they don't... think about just how much better you *could* be if you had *Boundless Energy.*

Well, the good news is that there *are* ways. Lots of small ways in fact that you can increase your energy levels and upgrade your health, fitness, brain power and more.

Let's start with your diet...

Your Energy Level Relates Directly to Your Diet

Diet is one of the biggest contributing factors to low energy –
both for the population in general and for individuals
specifically.

In the wild we would have eaten a diet that provided us with
tons of energy and that fueled us to chase down prey and to
generally perform at our optimum. It is not a coincidence that
the food available to us provided us with so much energy:
rather, our bodies evolved as they did *because* that was the
food that was around. In other words, through thousands of
years of evolution, we adapted to thrive on what was
available to us…

And now we're ruining it by surviving on a diet that contains
none of that goodness (or at least barely any).

Our Low Density, Simple Carb Diets

If you're like a lot of people, then you will come home from
work after a long, tiring day and you will throw on a pizza or
a microwave meal. Perhaps you'll have a piece of pie and
some chips.

Let's take a look at what you actually get from that.

Well, on an energy front you *do* get a lot of calories. In fact, a
standard shop-bought pie will normally land you about
600Kcal. Then you have the chips, which will add in another
200Kcal, your drink, your desert…

By the end, you've no doubt eaten over 1,000 calories, which happens to be half of most people's daily allowance (2,000 is a good average to follow here). This is what's making us fat and lugging all that extra bodyweight around with you is unsurprisingly a surefire way to make yourself tired.

Dumping that much food into your gut at once is also not a great move. Now you have a ton of food to process, including low-quality protein, which will slowly move through your digestive system robbing your other functions of energy.

What's more though, the calories you just took in were 'simple carbs'. The pastry around that pie, the chips, the desert, the drink – all of these are simple sugars that spike the blood stream immediately. And that's before you even count all the *added* sugar. Suddenly hitting your body with that much raw energy might sound like a *good* thing for your energy but in fact you couldn't be further from the truth. Instead, you're spiking your blood sugar, leading to a sudden surge of insulin and a 'high'. That insulin uses up the sugar and removes it from your blood but because you're not using it that quickly, it simply gets stored as fat (a process called lipogenesis). And guess how you feel once that process has ended? Exhausted! And you get a sudden energy slump (which by the way, is when most of us snack on *more* sugar).

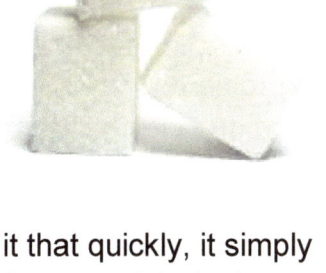

Worse yet, all those calories and simple carbs have done you approximately *zero* good. Why? Because they're such low quality. When you eat a shop-bought pie, unless you're spending lots of money, you're actually eating cuts of meat that are 'all the leftovers' blended together. All the pastry consists of is flour and sugar, the chips offer no nutritious value and everything you're eating has been preserved, transported and stored.

So all you're doing every night is dumping your body full of low-quality food to process and in vast quantities. Is it a wonder you wake up tired?

Supplements That Provide Energy

Now, I could tell you to cut it out. To stop eating that garbage and to start eating healthily again.

But it wouldn't do any good.

How can I be sure of that? Because you already *knew* that your diet probably wasn't all that healthy. You already *know* that home-cooked fresh ingredients are much better.

The problem? You don't have the time, energy or perhaps even money to change the way you eat. Notice that energy is a problem here: something of a vicious circle isn't it?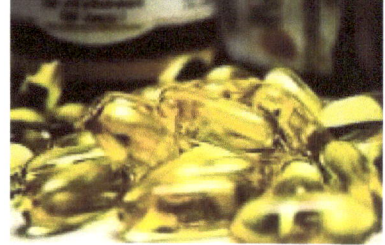

So to 'jumpstart' your self-improvement and your drive towards more energy, why don't we start with a supplement stack?

The following ingredients are things you can take with your meals which will greatly enhance your energy levels:

Vitamin D

Vitamin D is excellent for two things: improving your sleep and helping you to produce more testosterone. The vast majority of us are deficient, so take this in the morning and you'll start feeling a lot better.

Iron and Vitamin B12

Vitamin B12 and iron are required to give us our healthy red blood cells. In case you forgot, red blood cells are the oxygen-carrying portion of our blood which our body uses to burn fat and fuel all kinds of processes in our body.

Coconut Oil

Coconut oil is super 'in vogue' right now on the web and it deserves all the praise it's getting. Apart from being excellent for all kinds of beauty treatments, coconut oil contains medium-chain triglycerides which are a type of fat that stimulate the liver to produce ketones. If you've ever heard of a 'ketogenic diet', you'll know that ketones provide the body (and particularly the brain) with an alternate source of energy that it can't get from carbs.

Omega 3 Fatty Acid

Omega 3 fatty acid is an essential fatty acid that the body uses to create cell walls. This increases your 'cell membrane permeability' which is a very important value. Why? Because it helps the cells to communicate with one another and it allows neurotransmitters to pass more easily between brain cells.

Creatine

Creatine is a supplement used by athletes. Its job is to take the broken-down form of ATP (adenosine triphosphate) and recombine it for extra use in the body. What does this mean? Well, ATP is the main 'energy currency' of all life. It comes from glucose and releases energy when the bonds connecting three molecules are broken apart. This results in ADP (adenosine diphosphate) and AMP (adenosine monophosphate) – a two and a one. Normally that's all the use you can get out of it but with creatine, you are able to reuse the energy by rebonding the ADP and AMP back together.

The body produces creatine naturally but if you take it in supplement form you can get a little more. In real-terms this means a few extra seconds of exertion when lifting weights or running a marathon – and it means better mental energy for performing erythematic and fighting stress.

Lutein

Lutein is generally thought of as a supplement for the eyes to help prevent macular degeneration. In recent studies, it was found that it could also enhance the performance of the mitochondria – the energy factories that live inside each of our cells. When given to mice, it was found that they would voluntarily run miles further each week on their treadmills – pointing to increased energy and performance.

Garlic Extract

Garlic is a vasodilator. This means that it can widen the blood vessels to allow more blood and oxygen to get around – to the brain and muscles for instance - thus fueling you with more energy.

Vitamin B6

Vitamin B6 is used to help us extract energy from carbohydrates. At the same time, it is also used for the creation of neurotransmitters which helps it to boost cognitive performance. Low levels of B6 have been shown to result in lack of energy and focus and even shrinking brain tissue and Alzheimer's.

Coenzyme Q10

Coenzyme Q10 is another substance that athletes are very interested in at the moment and which can considerable increase the efficiency of the mitochondria for enhanced fat burning and energy production.

The Perfect Diet

Now that's a *lot* of different supplements to be taking. It's quite a long shopping list and it would get pretty expensive. If you can only afford a few, then I would recommend:

- Vitamin D

- Vitamin B6

- Garlic extract

- Omega 3 fatty acid

Here's the thing though: you actually *needn't* be taking *any* of these supplements. Not if your diet is correct.

All of these things can be found in your diet if you know where to look. CoQ10 and creatine are found in red meats, vitamins and minerals are found in all our fruits and vegetables, omega 3 fatty acid is found in fish, lutein is found in eggs…

If you just make sure that everything you're eating is fresh and nutritious, then you'll be providing your body with all the energy it needs. You'll be able to absorb it better and you'll be getting it in the right ratios and quantities. Ratios and quantities that you *evolved* to thrive on. Meanwhile, many other substances found in your diet can help to boost your energy levels too: zinc, magnesium, vitamin C, PQQ, l-carnitine, l-theanine, resveratrol… Eating a healthy diet is like having an incredibly expensive athlete's supplement stack! Only delicious…

Meanwhile, you should try to avoid the 'simple' carbs. That's anything that tastes sweet (like cake) and anything white (like pasta or rice). Instead, start eating brown rice and pasta, vegetables, spinach and have that in the place of your chips (as a rule, try to avoid processed, man-made carbs that you couldn't find). This will release energy much more slowly and provide you with a steady supply throughout the day. Don't be afraid of fat either – it contains more calories (9 per gram versus 4) but it's slow release too. Try to eat smaller portions, more often and don't over-stuff yourself.

How do you go about cooking these nutritious, fresh meals when you're so pushed for time and energy? Using the supplement stack can be a good head start but another tip is to prepare your meals at the start of the week.

Cook up a few pots of food you can dip into throughout the week and keep what you don't eat in the freezer or in a plastic contains.

On Going too Far...

If you've read much on diets before, then you might have noticed that this recommendation is somewhat close to the paleo diet and the slow carb diet.

Well, that's because *it is*… But we've stopped just short of going too far in either direction.

We eat too many processed carbs. Of that there's no doubt. And if we ate less of those carbs, we'd feel *much better*. At the same time though, we still need carbs. They're still an important food group in our diet and if we get the right kind in the right quantities, they actually boost testosterone production and aid with our general levels of energy and wellbeing. Restrict carbs too much and you'll feel tired. The occasionally bit of brown pasta with your bolognaise *won't kill you*. And the Chinese show that rice isn't terrible for your waistline! (In fact a lot of classic bodybuilders eat nothing but rice and steamed chicken)

Likewise, while natural, unprocessed foods are definitely healthier than cake, pie and chips, you don't need to eat 'only' the things you would find in the wild. A lot of serious paleo dieters will tell you not to eat bread, wheat or cheese. And they will *never* break their diet to have a bowl of pasta.

But here's the thing: most of the top performing athletes in

the world have performed just *fine* on bread (and you can forget about gluten being an issue unless you have an intolerance). Some of the smartest thinkers in the world drank lots of tea and ate lots of chocolate…

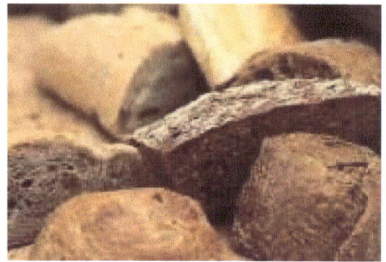

Point being? You can perform just fine eating a relatively 'normal' diet. And actually, our lifestyle places different demands on our body these days anyway, it's only natural our diet should adapt. So in other words, don't waste your energy thinking you can *only* eat specific foods. Just stick with your *current* diet but make it a little healthier by cutting back on the simple carbs and by injecting some more nutrients.

Habits and Lifestyle Effects Your Energy Levels Too

Once you've upgraded your diet, you'll find that you immediately start feeling more energetic. This is a *big* part of the battle. But really to improve your energy, you need to look at the bigger picture. No part of our health exists in a vacuum and even the best diet in the world can be undermined with the wrong lifestyle or the wrong routine.

In fact, you're probably doing a bunch of things right now that are completely ruining your energy levels. If you can just find these 'black holes' then you'll be able to save yourself large packets of energy to use in other, more constructive ways throughout the day…

Alcohol and Your Energy

Here comes the bad news: alcohol is very bad for your energy levels. As in, it's awful…

In the short term, alcohol is terrible for your energy and can leave you completely exhausted. The reason for that is that alcohol is actually a depressant. That means that it works to inhibit the firing of neurons in your brain, slowing down your thinking and making you sleepy. Alcohol, like a sleeping tablet or anxiolytic, works in the 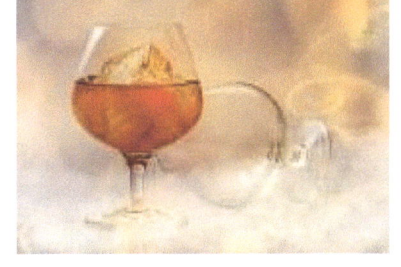 *opposite* manner to a stimulant. And because it causes whole brain areas to stop working, it can rob you of your higher order brain function too.

So if you were planning on being productive this evening – doing a workout, finishing some work – think twice about picking up that beer. At the same time, drinking beer also has longer-term knock-on effects on your energy levels and general health. Of course alcohol also contributes to weight gain at seven calories per gram. It causes headaches the next day and it significantly impairs the quality of your sleep Try wearing a heartrate monitor when you drink alcohol and you'll see it sends it sky-high, which isn't exactly conducive to a restful night! Although alcohol is a depressant, it 'amps up' the body as it tries to purge what is essentially a toxin from your system.

If you're going to enjoy alcohol though, try to have your last glass a few hours *before* bed. And try eating banana and honey sandwiches as a hangover cure. These work wonders as they line the stomach, replenish your energy stores, fix your electrolytes and break down acetaldehyde – a toxic substance that is responsible for a lot of the negative effects associated with hangover.

Water

So you shouldn't be drinking alcohol. What you *should* be drinking though is *water*.

Water is absolutely crucial to your energy levels as it's what the body uses for pretty much every crucial function. You've probably read stats telling you that your body is 70% water or there about and it's true – you are *mostly* water.

Too bad then that the majority of the US population are chronically dehydrated! This then leads to headaches, cramps, dry throats and of course – tiredness.

How much water should you be drinking? A good guide is to try and consume at least 7-10 glasses a day. Try this and you should find that you start feeling *much* more human if you weren't doing it already.

Sitting Too Much

If you work an office job, then the simple fact of the matter is that you probably sit *far* too much. Even if you *don't* have an office job but you like to spend your evenings relaxing in front of the television: you almost certainly sit too much as well.

Sitting is bad for us for all kinds of reasons. The main one though is that it's terrible for our hearts – the longer you spend sitting during the day, the more likely you are to die young – and the main reason for that is that your heart health declines.

Think about your dog or your cat. They are typically either very active, chasing things around the house, going for long walks etc. or they are sleeping. Most animals, when left to their own devices, do not just sit statically for long periods of time – and neither should you!

Thus, if you are spending a lot of time just sitting down, there's a very good chance that your heart is weakening and your fitness is less than it could be. And you might even be shortening your lifespan.

And most of us don't sit with particularly good posture. In fact, there *isn't* really a good posture for sitting and however you try to position yourself you're likely to cause some damage.

The main problem is that your legs are lifted up at right angles. This is a very 'scrunched up' position to be in and is pretty much the opposite of a stretch. Thus, the muscles on the tops of your legs that help you lift your leg up (a group known as the hip flexors), will become shorter and tighter over time if you sit a lot. Meanwhile, the muscles on the *backs* of your legs that bring your thighs back down (the hip extensors) will become elongated, stretched and weak (and it doesn't help that you're sitting on your hamstrings and glutes all day either).

Likewise, your arms will be forward in a typing position, which will shorten your pecs and weaken your back muscles. You'll be looking downwards towards the computer and your shoulders will likely be hunched. All of this leads to condition known as 'kyphosis' where you have a permanent hunch.

These problems with your biomechanics can then lead to a number of other issues. Common for instance is to get neck pain and headaches. Likewise, you might find that you get pain in the small of your back and that you struggle to bend down to pick things up.

And what you might not realize is just how much your energy levels and mood can be impacted by poor flexibility. You can then find yourself struggling to do simple things, aching when you wake up in the mornings and generally struggling to get around and move normally – you can feel prematurely like an elderly man or woman! Imagine if you could move your joints more freely, if you didn't have nagging pains and if your fitness was improved? All this could be fixed by just sitting a little less.

But you probably aren't sitting all day for the fun of it. More likely, you work the job you do because you need the money and because you don't have another option. Here are some tips that can help then:

- Ensure you have the proper posture at work – keep your computer monitor head height so you aren't looking down and have your arms at right angles. Bring your keyboard in nearer to you.

- Look for a supportive chair.

- Change position occasionally – if you have the option to, take a laptop to different parts of your working area.

- If that's not an option, then just make sure that you're getting up and moving around often. Take a ten minute break every hour or so and if you need to take a call, try pacing around the office while you take it.

- You can even consider looking into a standing desk. While it's hard to focus standing, you can at least stand up when answering e-mails or performing other tasks that don't require a lot of attention.

Stress Management

But if there is one thing about working in an office that is bad for your health and your energy levels, it would not be the way you're sitting. Far more destructive by far is stress, which is something that a great many of us experience in the work place. If you are very stressed at work, then you should not underestimate just what a severe impact this can have on your health, your mood and your energy levels.

The reason that we as humans get stressed is that in the wild, it would have helped us to survive dangerous situations. The idea of stress is to increase our awareness, our physical strength and our ability to think quickly. Thus, when we are stressed, our bodies respond by releasing dopamine, norepinephrine and other 'fight or flight' hormones. This increases our heartrate; it directs more blood flow to the muscles and to the brain and it heightens our awareness. At the same time, we might start trembling, our immune systems and digestive systems will be suppressed and we'll feel anxious and jittery.

All these effects are designed to help us in a combat or escape situation. In other words, they are meant to come on fast and be over quickly. If we saw a predator or prey, if we had a fight with someone, or if we saw a fire – then this would be exactly how the fight or flight 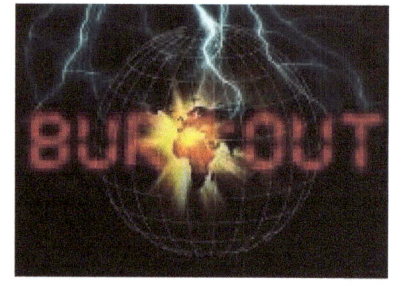 system would work and it would probably help us to stay alive.

Today though, stress is not acute – it is chronic. Our modern sources of stress include things like angry bosses, poor finances, strained relationships, looming deadlines… all these are things that have no finite end, or no *imminent* end at least. In other words, our body is *constantly* in this state of arousal and as such, our immune system is constantly suppressed leaving us susceptible to illness. Likewise, so too is our digestion, robbing us of the nutrients we *should* be getting from our food. We'll also feel anxious and jittery and this will prevent us from sleeping well.

And eventually, the brain will 'run low' on those fight or flight hormones. At this point, your sympathetic nervous system burns out and you reach a point known as 'adrenal fatigue'. It's then that you will find yourself robbed of the neurotransmitters that normally help you to get up in the morning and to focus on the task in hand. And without these neurotransmitters, you will feel demotivated, low on energy and listless – it is even correlated with depression.

So if you're getting to that point where you have no energy in the morning and where it's all just starting to feel a little bit too hard to carry on – you're probably experiencing adrenal fatigue as a result of stress.

If you *are* in that situation, then it's highly advisable that you change some aspect of your lifestyle or your routine. While it might not be easy to quit your job, to take time out of a relationship, or to speak to a financial advisor – it's crucial that you do. Ultimately, your health and your quality of life are what you should be putting first above *all* else. So if something is causing you a lot of stress and there's *anything* you can do about it… you should act.

If not, then you have some other options. One is to simply take some time off – having a holiday for instance. Another is to ask for help and to speak with friends about your stress. You'd be surprised what a big help it can be just to speak about your problems.

Finally, consider getting therapy from a cognitive behavioral therapist. This type of therapy is a very grounded and 'results focused' form of therapy that teaches you specific tools for dealing with mental health problems like stress.

CBT uses tools and techniques that allow you to exactly pinpoint what precisely it is making you stressed in the first place (a process called 'mindfulness') and it uses techniques that you can use to assess just how bad the things you're stressed about really are. Most often you will find that when you really assess your fears and stresses logically, there's actually nothing to be afraid of. Sometimes getting over stress is just a case of facing your fears.

Poor Quality of Sleep Can Drain Energy Levels

What do you want to do when you feel really tired and you have no energy left to do anything?

You want to sleep, right?

This should tell you quite plainly how important sleep is for energy. In fact, sleep is something of a miracle cure for all kinds of ailments – it improves your memory, your focus, your attention, your mood and your sleep *immensely*. Sleeping is far more effective than any beauty treatment, any 'smart drug' and any supplement. Get the right sleep and you will perform on the top of your game the next day – it's that simple.

Most of us don't get the quality or the quantity of sleep that we need though and as such we find ourselves walking around like zombies. We're cranky, we're easily distracted, we're confused and generally we operate like shadows of our true selves.

So how do you go about upgrading your sleep and getting back your low energy levels? Especially in a world that is 'always on' and always on the go.

Tricks to Improve Your Sleep Quality

Take a quick cursory look online and you'll find that there are thousands of different tips and 'hacks' that can supposedly give us better sleep. Everyone it seems has some kind of tip that can lead to amazing sleep and indeed there are a lot of good ones out there.

But again, some of them involve a lot of work and very little pay off. So instead, let's focus on the best ones that really make a noticeable difference and that are relatively easy to perform.

The good news is that if you're following the tips in this book so far, you should *already* find yourself sleeping much better. That's because you'll have more energy from more efficient mitochondria – and studies show that this is actually crucial for sleep. It's again something of a vicious cycle: but low energy leads to poor sleep and poor sleep leads to lower energy!

Likewise, if you're eating healthier you'll be getting the vitamin D, the zinc and magnesium and all kinds of other important nutrients to help your body recover through the night. Finally, if you're reducing your stress, you'll find that this *massively* has an impact on your ability to sleep as you'll be able to much more easily 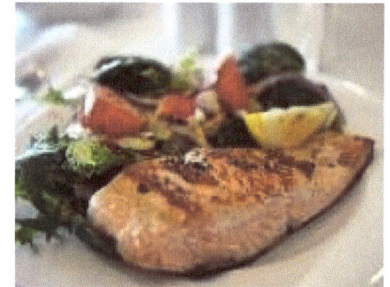 switch off from the stresses of the day.

At the same time, try these additional strategies:

Take a Hot Bath or Shower Before Bed

This is one of the most powerful ways to help yourself sleep more deeply. Taking a hot shower just before you go to sleep will not only relax your muscles, it will also trigger your body to produce growth hormone and melatonin, essentially getting you nicely drowsy.

Have Half an Hour to Rest Before Bed

If there's 'one life hack' that absolutely *everyone* should subscribe to these days, it's this one. No matter what else is going on in your life: take half an hour before bed to read a book and to relax. Keep your phone off and have just a dim bedside lamp. Don't watch TV and generally let yourself treat this like a 'wind down' time.

What this does is to allow you to forget the stresses of the day and to feel more relaxed as a result. Moreover, the lack of 'screen time' means that your brain will be able to begin producing more melatonin. When you look at a computer or TV screen, your brain interprets the wavelength of the light as being sunlight. As a result, it acts as though it is daytime and it floods your body with cortisol, preventing you from sleeping.

And this is why it's *also* so important to make sure there's no light on in your room.

Seriously though, the benefits of having half an hour to yourself to unwind go far beyond just better sleep. When your life is constantly rushed and you never have any time for 'you', it can often feel as though you're constantly being pushed to your limit. Start taking this time off to decompress and the world can seem a lot easier to manage.

Get Into a Routine

Something important to understand about the human body is that it works to rhythms. Your body likes routine because this allows it to learn natural rhythms – highs and lows that will stay consistent ensuring you start winding down biologically at the right moment.

This can make a big difference then to your ability to doze off and it will also allow you to control the amount of sleep you're getting more carefully. As you likely know, eight hours is a good ball-park figure to aim for if you can.

Likewise, you should also try to reserve your room purely for sleeping and sex. This is important because it creates an association between your room and sleep. This way, when you head to your room, it will act like a trigger that tells your body it's bed time and you'll begin to feel drowsy almost right away!

Perfect Your Environment

These are the 'easy tips' that pretty much everyone already knows about sleeping – but they're important and so they're still very much worth going over.

So another key thing to look at to make sure you're sleeping optimally is your environment, which must be:

- Completely silent

- As pitch black as possible

- Clean (if possible)

- Comforting

If you struggle to maintain a tidy room, or if you don't have much control over things like the amount of light, then a good strategy is just to get a curtain to go around your bed. That way you can block out the light and give yourself a private space *within* your larger room even.

Obvious it's also very important to wear comfortable pajamas (or sleep naked, which is currently preferred by the research), to invest in a comfortable bed (one of the best purchases you will ever make) and to keep your room the right temperature. The ideal temperature is for your room to be a little bit cool, which is again how we are evolutionarily designed to sleep.

How to Calm Your Mind

But what if you're someone who *can't* sleep? What if your mind is constantly active and you lie in bed with it racing, unable to switch off?

This is a problem a lot of people face and it can severely rob them of their energy levels the next day. And actually *that* is the problem.

You see, when you lie in bed and try to sleep, you might find that it actually *makes you stressed*. The fear of *not* getting to sleep, or the frustration and the expectation, are so great that they actually cause you to lie awake worrying. Ever had that 'hot and bothered' feeling where you look at the clock, see it says 4am and then curse the world for being able to sleep when you cannot?

This isn't exactly how you sink off to sleep!

To get around this problem then, we're going to once again take a leaf out of the CBT book (cognitive behavioral therapy). The idea then, is to change the way you approach sleep and the way you think about it. Specifically, you're going to stop pressuring yourself to sleep and to instead just allow yourself to relax. Consider sleep to be a bonus.

So tell yourself that it's fine to just relax in bed and to enjoy being comfy – because it *is*. That's good for you too. You can't force yourself to sleep, so don't try. Just lie there and enjoy not having to do anything, enjoy not having to be anywhere and enjoy the feeling of closing your eyes and listening to your breathing.

What you'll find, quite ironically, is that as soon as you start taking this approach… you drift right off!

Should You Power Nap?

With the best will in the world, there will still be times when you don't have the very best sleep and when all your sleeping strategies fail you. In those scenarios, what do you do? Well, one good strategy is just to *try again later*.

Remember when we compared your energy levels to those of your cat or dog? We said that the cat and dog were either active, or asleep – never anything in between. You can do the same thing yourself by sleeping throughout the day to catch up on some shuteye and many studies have shown that this can boost productivity, mood and more.

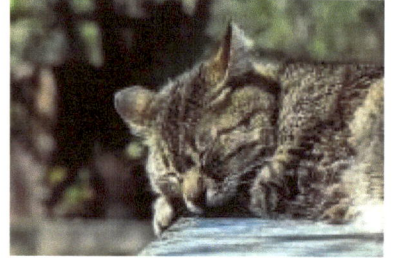

So how do you nap correctly? The secret is to time it correctly and specifically to aim to nap for around 90 minutes, not more and not less. This is important because of the way our body cycles through different stages of sleep (the body loves rhythms remember!). In 90 minutes you will go through one complete sleep cycle and will go from the lightest stage of sleep, to SWS (slow wave sleep) to REM.

You'll then be woken up just as you start to come around. On the other hand, you can sleep for 10-20 minutes in order to wake up *before* you go into the deeper stages of sleep and to avoid sleep inertia that way. 90 minutes is definitely better though, as dreaming is considered to be instrumental in helping us lay down new memories and boost our performance.

Is Your Morning Routine Helping or Hurting Your Energy Level?

In the last chapter we looked at how to get off to sleep and how to ensure we sleep well. That's one part of the story but what comes next is *waking up* the next day. How do you ensure you can spring out of bed and get lots done?

How to Wake Up Full of Energy

Now you know how to get to sleep, the next question is how you wake *up*. This is the key piece of the puzzle that most people overlook when it comes to sleeping well – but having a good night's sleep does not *necessarily* mean you'll be able to wake up easily too!

Too many of us wake up feeling groggy, lethargic and tired and as a result we waste the first half of the day. Some of us will even feel very sick in the morning, or have bad headaches.

If you fall into this latter category, then of course this is not normal, should not be considered 'okay' and is something you should look into. A few common culprits for feeling sick, headachey or 'coldy' in the morning include:

Dehydration – Try drinking a large glass of water before bed and you won't wake up with a dry throat or headache.

Low blood sugar – When you go to sleep, you are essentially fasting for 8 hours straight without food. As a result, you can feel sick when you wake up.

There are some theorists who even believe that this is why we have grown to eat desert as the last meal of the day! Some people recommend having a teaspoon of honey before bed to provide a steady flow of sugar (sucrose and fructose) throughout the night.

Mold – If you have mold in your room this can leave you feeling ill owing to the mycotoxins that it releases. Other signs of mold include a musky smell and damp air. If you notice these things, it can be worth getting a remediation company in – even if you can't see mold it can sometimes be building up underneath the floorboards or behind the paint in your rooms!

Allergies – If you're waking up hoarse with a headache, then allergies are a common cause. Even if you don't think you have any allergies, remember that they can come on at any point during your lifetime and as such you may have *developed* hay fever or similar.

Sleep Apnea – Sleep apnea is a condition that causes you to wake up for brief spells during the night because you've stopped breathing. In some cases this is due to a blocked passage (obstructive apnea) but in others it may have no cause (primary apnea). The best way to diagnose this is to film yourself sleeping, ask a friend to watch you, or potentially visit a sleep clinic. Either way, you might be prescribed a CPAP (continuous positive airway pressure) device which can prevent the problem.

If you address all these factors then you *should* find you start feeling much fresher and more energetic in the morning.

Something else that can help is to look into getting a 'daylight lamp'. These are lamps that emit a light wave very similar to the sun and which will gradually get brighter in the morning. This can help to *gradually* nudge you out of a deep sleep rather than waking you in the deepest stages of sleep. At the same time, these lamps can help to combat mild cases of 'SAD' (seasonal affective disorder) which is a condition that leaves people feeling tired, lethargic and even potentially depressed during the darker winter months. It can also help to put your biological clock more in-sync with your routine and in general it's a very useful tool for waking up more gradually and naturally – it's certainly much better than being startled out of your sleep by a blaring alarm clock.

And another trick you can use that's slightly controversial for waking up in the morning is to use your phone. A lot of people will tell you *not* to use your phone in the morning to get up but if you're someone who struggles to wake up in the morning it can actually be useful. The idea here is to set yourself to receive something you're looking forward to in the morning – subscribe to some good RSS feeds for instance, or join a community on a subject you're interested. What this does then is give you a motivation to sit up just a *little* first thing in the morning to grab your phone. If you can motivate yourself to do just that little bit and to start reading, you'll find that you gradually come around.

Finally, you might also consider using a fitness tracking device that offers sleep tracking. A great example of this would be the Jawbone UP. This device has a great feature which is to wake you up out of a light sleep by watching your movement during the night. You set an alarm – say for 7am – and it waits for a moment *near then* when you're in light sleep rather than deep sleep.

It might go off at 6.30 for instance, or 6.45 but never after 7am. What this means is you're now waking up out of light sleep instead of a heavy sleep which helps to prevent 'sleep inertia'. In theory, you should be much more awake.

Sleep trackers can be great for improving energy in other ways too. While the Microsoft Band lacks this particular feature, it also has a constant heartrate monitor which allows you to measure your heartrate throughout the night. This gives a much more accurate measure of your sleep as well as your calories burned and that in turn will allow you to run experiences to see which sleeping strategies are the most effective for helping you get proper restoration.

What to do First?

So now you're out of bed, what do you do first? A healthy breakfast is a great start to your day and a coffee if you're so inclined (though in the long term, caffeine actually does more harm than good to energy levels).

Using the tips above you should be feeling fairly awake but with the best will in the world, you'll still potentially feel a little groggy in the morning sometimes and need a bit of help waking up.

One thing that can *really* help you to wake up then, is to take a cold shower. A cold shower will not only shock you into wakefulness, it will actually trigger the release of norepinephrine and dopamine thus making you more alert and even speed up your metabolism to burn more fat. As a way to wake up, this beats a cup of coffee any day!

Next you'll probably have to commute into work. This is actually one of the very worst things for many of us when it comes to stress and energy. Not only is it stressful sitting in traffic or on a busy train but it's also a waste of energy. What's more, if you walk on busy streets in the morning, your body will view this as the equivalent of being leapt out on repeatedly by hundreds of people. Did you know that 'things moving toward us' is the *only* universal fear that we all share? This can drastically raise your heartrate and make you feel really rather exhausted when you get into work.

What's the solution? There's no easy one. Of course you should look for a less stressful commute if possible but at the very least just keep it in mind when thinking about your energy and stress levels.

Then, when starting your working day, remember that you're not performing at your absolute optimum. A good type of work to begin with is something that you can do relatively 'mindlessly'. A mindless job is anything that you could perform equally well with the TV on.

Affect Your Energy Level Through Exercise

When we feel low on energy, exercise can often feel like the last thing we want to do. In fact though, exercising is one of *the* most powerful ways to boost energy levels in both the very short term *and* the much longer term.

In this chapter, we'll look at precisely how exercise does this and at what kind of exercise does it best.

How Exercise Improves Your Energy

Short Term

In the short term, exercise can give you a great energy boost which is why it's a good way to start your day. If you're wondering about that commute quandary in the previous chapter, consider jogging or cycling into work!

One reason that exercising is so good for you in the short term is that it encourages healthy circulation. Exercise gets your heart beating which sends more blood to your muscles and to your brain. That means more oxygen and more nutrients which is essentially like getting an injection of rocket fuel!

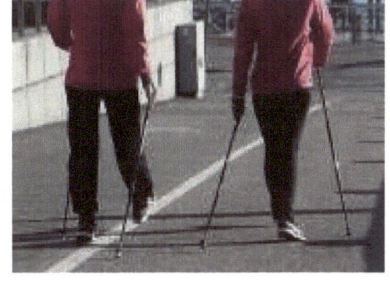

Exercise *also* stimulates the release of lots of very positive hormones and neurotransmitters. If you've heard of the 'runners' high' then you should know that jogging can stimulate the release of endorphins and serotonin. The result is that you feel very positive, very happy and of course very high in energy.

As an added bonus, exercise is also one of *the* most potent ways to boost the restorative nature of your sleep (we saved this one!). When you workout during the day, you will burn much more energy which will mean you're far readier to doze off at night – especially if you got lots of fresh air by working out outside.

Long Term

But the long term benefits of exercise are *much* more profound.

For starters, exercise will help you to burn calories and lose weight. This then means that again you'll be carrying less excess weight around with you and will feel lighter, nimbler and far more energetic as a result.

On top of this, exercise will also help to improve your fitness. This means a stronger heart and a better VO2 max. What this refers to is your body's ability to bring in oxygen and to utilize it for energy in a short space of time. A high VO2 max means that you can run long distances without panting and feeling out of breath. This also just so happens to be the perfect antidote to all that sitting...

And if you can run a marathon without feeling out of breath then imagine how much easier that walk to work or that hike up the stairs will be!

Exercise also builds muscle and believe it or not, that too can help you to feel more energetic. The main reason for this is that it makes various activities less strenuous and tiring – if you've built strong muscles then you'll find lifting things much easier, walking much easier and... pretty much everything else much easier too!

Better yet, exercise can also boost your mitochondrial count. As you'll hopefully remember from *various* points throughout this book, your mitochondria are the energy centers of your cells that help you to utilize ATP and to power yourself through your day. In fact, going back to another early observation (about children seeming to have limitless energy) it is thought that we get more tired as we get older because our mitochondria stop functioning properly.

Exercise increases the quantity and efficiency of mitochondria and especially when you use HIIT. HIIT is 'High Intensity Interval Training' and is a type of exercise that involves brief bursts of exertion lasting a couple of minutes, followed by longer bursts of 'active recovery'.

So while some exercise programs might have you running on a treadmill for 10 minutes at 50% of your maximum capacity, a HIIT workout would involve *sprinting* on a treadmill for two minutes, then power walking for three and then sprinting for another two minutes. This type of exercise has been shown to be more efficient in a shorter time span and is generally a great way to give yourself a boost mentally and physically.

How to Train

Using HIIT is a very good idea then if you want to get the most energy benefit from your training. You should also combine this with some weight lifting in order to get the benefit of more physical strength (and actually, weight lifting is very good for weight loss and improving your metabolism).

What's also important though, is to avoid *over doing* your training. This is the big mistake that a lot of people make when taking on any new workout routine and it can end up being almost as bad as *not* exercising at all.

If you lift weights until you are sore for instance, then just bear in mind that this now means you're going to be sore for the rest of that day and probably for the next *two* days. What's the point of being at your physical best if you hurt every time you move? Likewise, if you run too far and too fast, you'll end up feeling too weak and low on energy for the following days and nights. Continue this over-exertion too long and it can eventually lead to 'overtraining' which leaves you feeling tired, listless and upset.

Something to pay attention to here is your 'heartrate variance'. This shows you how well recovered you are after a workout in the morning and while it's hard to measure this without a piece of hardware, measuring your grip strength *can* provide something of an indication. Most important is to train to the point where it's still fun, to push yourself but not too hard and to *listen* to what your body is telling you.

Synchronize Your Work With Your High Energy Level

Using all the advice we've covered so far in this book, you should now be reaching the point where you are somewhat the 'master' of your own energy and able to increase it significantly. Even with this knowledge though, it's important to realize that you still aren't *completely* in charge of your energy levels and you're still in some ways a slave to higher forces.

Specifically, you are a slave to those natural rhythms we talked about. Your energy levels ebb and flow like waves and at some points you are going to be high in energy and at other points you are going to be *low* in energy. This is set partly by your internal body clock (internal pacemaker) and partly by external cues (external zeitgebers) such as social cues, eating habits and light.

In the morning when you wake up, your body is flooded with cortisol and this helps you to start shifting into first gear. Your energy then remains fairly steady until lunch, when you replenish your glucose stores and then again at 4pm at which point you will reach a low point in your natural energy cycle. 4pm is when many of us start feeling sleepy and wanting to curl up on the couch. We also feel more tired straight after food while we're digesting, so if you eat lunch at 3.30pm, you may as well write 4pm off completely.

Your energy will improve after 4pm but will slowly tail off until bed time. There will be another slump, peak and slump following dinner.

Structuring Your Day for Optimum Productivity

Simply knowing that these ebbs and flows exist and knowing when you're going to be performing your best can help a great deal with your ability to stay productive and to get the most out of yourself.

For instance, if you have flexible working hours (or a reasonable boss), consider speaking with them and asking if you can move your working day forward one hour. Get into work at 8 when your energy will be on the rise and then leave at 4pm when you'll be starting to 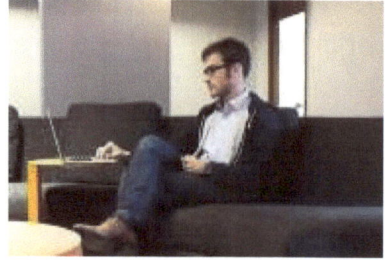 struggle focusing. You can then let your energy continue to sink as you relax for the evening.

Another tip is to avoid having big plans after dinner. If you have anything productive to do, then do it *before* you eat. The minute you eat dinner and sit on the couch, your energy will be in decline and you should consider the productive part of the day over.

This also applies on a larger scale. Specifically, you will find that you also have months where you are more productive and months where you are less so. This is particularly true when it comes to exercise – you can have months of being highly disciplined and training well and then often find they're followed by months of not having the energy. Don't punish yourself for this, just go with your body's natural inclination and try to plan tasks for the points in time when you are most likely to be able to focus on and complete them.

Individual Differences and How to Control Your Cycles

We've looked at the times you're most likely to be productive or sleepy during the day and for most people this should ring true. Do keep in mind though that everyone is different. Some people are night owls and actually are more productive later at night, while other people are 'early birds' and will tend to get their best work done first thing in the morning when the rest of us are still groggy and experiencing sleep inertia. Try to learn your own individual rhythms and work with those.

At the same time, remember as well that you *can* actually control your rhythms in order to help your energy cycles sync up with what you're doing at any given time. The daylight lamp we mentioned earlier is one and another is to time when you eat carefully. Not only can changing your eating schedule help you move that after-dinner slump, it also actually affects your body clock. Eat dinner later and you'll find it a little easier to sleep later. Daytime naps can also help with this.

Now It's All Up to You ...

Throughout the course of this book we've covered a lot of different points and right now your mind might be swimming with ideas for how to get more energy and how to change your routine for the better.

To help you cement all these ideas then, let's quickly recap on some of the tools and strategies you can now be using to get more energy:

- Start eating more healthily

    o Avoid processed foods

    o Avoid simple carbohydrates

    o Eat nutrient dense foods

    o Eat smaller meals, more regularly

    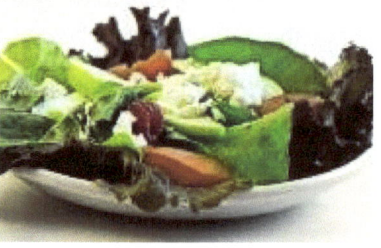

    o Eat complex carbs that release energy more slowly

    o Don't get too carried away with fad diets

    o Prepare meals in advance

    o Supplement if necessary

- Exercise more

    o Use HIIT training to increase mitochondria

- o Don't over train

- Manage your sleep

  - o Have half an hour to relax in the evenings

  - o Take a hot shower before bed

  - o Sleep with the window ajar

  - o Invest in comfortable bedclothes and pajamas

- Wake up slowly

  - o Use a daylight alarm

  - o And sleep tracker

  - o Tempt yourself out of bed with something interesting

  - o Take a cold shower!

  - o Cycle or jog to work if you can

- Plan your day to coincide with your natural energy highs and lows

  - o Ask if you can start an hour earlier and finish at four

  - o Don't plan anything for after dinner – do productive things first

  - o Time meals to adjust your body clock

  - o Learn what works for you!

All of this might sound like quite a lot and especially if you're feeling low on energy. If you're exhausted right now, then can you *really* be bothered to take up a new exercise regime? To cycle to work? To change your whole routine? To cook fresh meals?

This might sound like a lot and it might sound daunting but that's why it can pay to keep in mind the principle of Kaizen. Kaizen means making small, incremental changes that all add up into something big and profound.

For instance then, try swapping your morning coffee for a smoothie and feel how much more energy you get from nutrients versus caffeine. It's a very small change but it makes a huge difference.

If you can't commit to half an hour of chilling in the evening, try making it ten minutes.

And if working out is too daunting, commit just to half an hour a week to begin with.

These small changes might not seem like much but just a little bit of extra energy can go a long way and ultimately will lead to a domino effect. By the end you'll feel brighter, you'll look healthier, you'll be happier, you'll work better…

And it all starts with you by making just one small lifestyle change…

Other Senior Health and Fitness Books by This Author

If you would like to read more about Senior Health and Fitness, here is a list of the <u>titles, CreateSpace links and descriptions:</u>

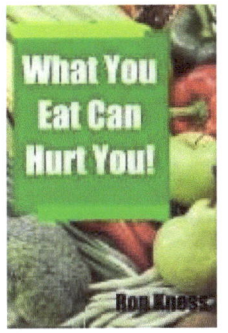

What You Eat Can Hurt You

https://www.createspace.com/4963196

Do you know that certain foods increase your risk for inflammation, disease and illness? It's true! And certain foods can help cure and heal you if you do get sick. Knowing which foods to eat and which ones to avoid empowers you to manage your own health.

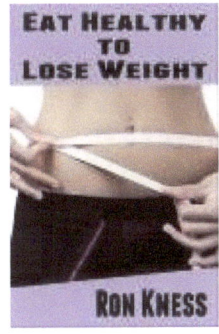

Eat Healthy to Lose Weight

https://www.createspace.com/4962939

As you read through our book, we show you which foods you should and should not be eating to reach your weight loss goal, along with discussing how to maintain your weight loss and stay within a few pounds of your goal weight. Banish the weight you keep gaining back each time by learning how to live a healthy lifestyle.

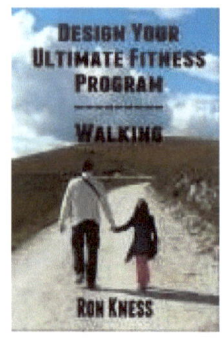

Design Your Ultimate Fitness Program - Walking

https://www.createspace.com/5252272

In my book Design Your Ultimate Fitness Program – Walking, we discuss the considerations that need to be made when designing a custom walking program, along with:

• Equipment needed
• Wearable technology you can use to track your walking
• And how to make walking more challenging

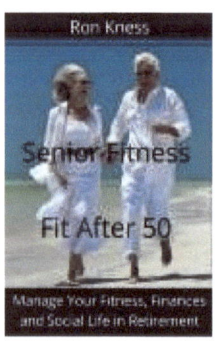

Senior Fitness – Fit After 50: Learn How to Manage Your Fitness, Finances and Social Life in Retirement

https://www.createspace.com/5474751

Inside you will discover answers to your most pressing questions:
• What do I need to know about downsizing my home?
• What are the best tips for staying healthy as you approach your 50's?
• When should I start planning for retirement?
• I am worried about being lonely once I retire, do others feel the same?
• Is it worthwhile to carry two homes during retirement?
And more…

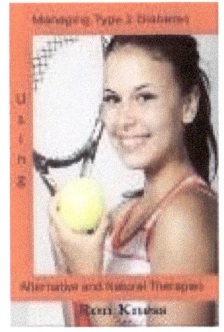

Managing Type 2 Diabetes Using Alternative And Natural Therapies

https://www.createspace.com/5401244

While Type 2 diabetes can be managed medically, there are many alternative natural and holistic methods of therapy and treatment that can further enhance quality of life and minimize the effects of this disease. In this book, I discuss 12 different types, including yoga, reflexology and acupuncture to name just three.

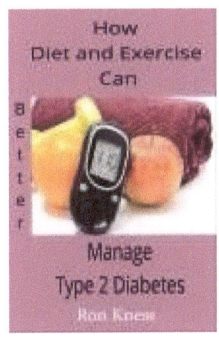

How Diet and Exercise Can Better Manage Type 2 Diabetes

https://www.createspace.com/5404845

Of the different types of diabetes, only Type 2 can be reversed. In my book How Diet and Exercise Can Better Manage Type 2 Diabetes, we reveal the three things you can do to best manage your disease, including:

• Diet
• Exercise
• Weight management

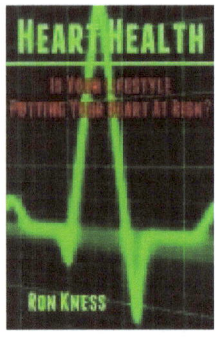

Heart Health: Is Your Lifestyle Putting Your Heart at Risk?

https://www.createspace.com/5464020

In my ebook Is Your Lifestyle Putting Your Heart At Risk? we discuss the six greatest risks to your heart and the lifestyle changes you can make to mitigate them.

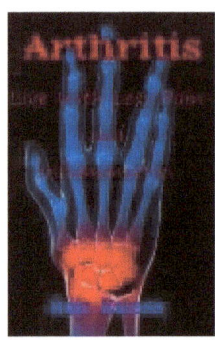

Arthritis – Live Wth Less Pain and Inflammation: Tips and Techniques You Can Use to Lessen the Pain and Inflammation

https://www.createspace.com/5457441

Discover Simple Tips & Information That Will Help Reduce The Painful Symptoms Of Arthritis!

You learn things like:
• Simple and effective information that will help you manage the pain and inflammation that comes along with arthritis, so that you can live an active, full life without debilitating pain.
• The different types of arthritis, their symptoms and how to alleviate their painful side effects.
• The pros and cons of over-the-counter arthritis medications, plus simple tips that will help you know how to choose the right supplements.
• Free, yet effective ways to get relief from arthritis pain and inflammation, so you don't have to suffer anymore.

The effects arthritis can have significant impact on your physical and mental well-being, but this books shows you how to overcome its painful symptoms and live life relatively pain free.

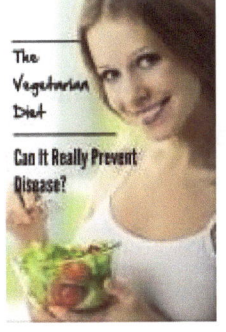

[The Vegetarian Diet – Can It Really Prevent Disease?](#)

https://www.createspace.com/5519874

Is a vegetarian diet right for you? Multiple studies have shown over and over that a vegetarian diet goes along way in preventing certain chronic diseases, such as:

• Heart Disease
• Cancer
• Diverticulitis
• Type 2 Diabetes
• Hypertension
• Obesity
• Kidney Failure

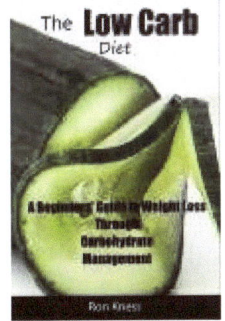

[The Low Carb Diet: A Beginner's Guide to Weight Loss Through Carbohydrate Management](#)

https://www.createspace.com/5416348

In my book "The Low-Carb Diet – A Beginners' Guide to Weight Loss Through Carbohydrate Management", I reveal a successful method of losing weight based in part on the amount and type of carbohydrates you consume.

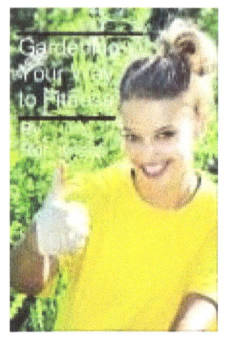

Gardening Your Way to Fitness: The Fun Way to Get Fit and Provide Beauty and Healthful Bounty for Your Family

https://www.createspace.com/5459564

The gym is a great place to stay fit during the colder seasons, but once the temperature turns warmer you want to spend more time outside. Plus, you'll have the benefit of fresh wholesome produce to enjoy by growing vegetables in your backyard garden.

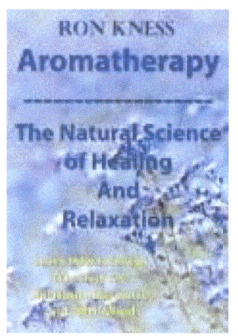

Aromatherapy - The Science of Healing and Relaxation: Learn How Essential Oils Elicit The Relaxation Response And Alter Mood

https://www.createspace.com/5714434

In my book Aromatherapy – The Science of Healing and Relaxation, we reveal the natural holistics methods you can use to heal the body from certain medical issues and to relive stress through relaxation. In particular we talk about:

• Aromatherapy - what it is and how it works
• Essential Oils – how the effects of certain aromas differs from others
• Recipes – how to make your own essential oil combinations

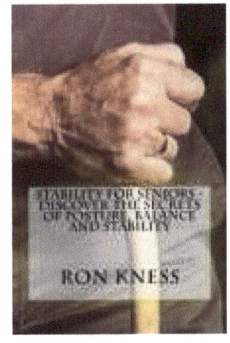

[Stability for Seniors](https://www.createspace.com/6096479): [Discover the Secrets of Posture, Balance and Stability](https://www.createspace.com/6096479)

https://www.createspace.com/6096479

Many people sacrifice their health in pursuit of their career. They are so busy making a living that they neglect to make a life. The excuse that they do not have time to exercise is tossed about so frequently that they end up letting their health and fitness slide.

If you are not regularly active, you will have muscular atrophy over time. Your flexibility will decrease. Your core strength will diminish. As time progresses, you will be less limber and more rigid.

This is exactly how people age poorly. It's a process that has snowballed over time.

Only with regular exercise and a healthy diet can you have a body that is fit and has the ability to almost reverse aging.

If you have neglected your health for years and life seems to be a chore now because you can't get around without assistance, do not feel dejected.

You can remedy the situation. You can restore the strength, balance and stamina that you have lost. It is never too late to become what you might have been.

This guide will show you exactly what you need to do to restore your balance, strengthen your core and give you the ability to live life to its fullest. Read how …

About the Author

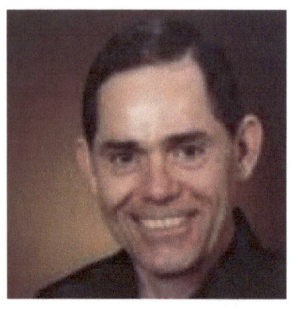

Ron Kness is an entrepreneur living in the U.S.A. who loves sharing knowledge and helping others on the topic of living a healthy lifestyle.

Ron is a passionate person who will go the extra mile and over-deliver.

His words of wisdom:

"I believe that knowledge is power. Everyone should improve themselves and/or business, no matter what stage in life they're in. Whether it's to develop a better mindset or to increase profits. Moving forward is key."

If you would like to learn more from Ron, please visit his website:

www.ingramcontent.com/pod-product-compliance
Lightning Source LLC
Chambersburg PA
CBHW050821290526
45792CB00001B/212